How to treat Impotence using Cialis Tadalafil Pills for Men

by:

Dr. Howard M. Barnes

Table of Contents

Introduction

Impotence, also known as erectile dysfunction (ED), is a condition that affects a significant number of men worldwide. Despite its prevalence, the topic often remains shrouded in stigma and misinformation. This article aims to shed light on the prevalence of impotence in men, exploring its incidence across various age groups, ethnicities, and geographical locations. By understanding the scope of the issue, we can better address the needs of those affected and work towards more effective treatments and interventions.

What is Impotence?

Before diving into the statistics, it's crucial to define what impotence or erectile dysfunction entails. ED is the inability to achieve or maintain an erection sufficient for sexual intercourse. The condition can be temporary or chronic, and its causes can be either psychological or physiological, or a combination of both.

Prevalence by Age

One of the most significant factors influencing the prevalence of impotence is age. While ED can affect men at any age, the likelihood increases significantly with age:

- Young Adults (18-30): Studies suggest that about 8-10% of men in this age group experience ED to some degree.
- Middle-Aged Men (31-60): The prevalence rises to approximately 40% in men aged 40 and above.
- Older Adults (61 and above): For men over 60, the prevalence can be as high as 60-70%.

Global Prevalence

Erectile dysfunction is a global issue, affecting men of all ethnicities and backgrounds. According to the Global Burden of Disease Study, an estimated 322 million men worldwide will experience ED by the year 2025, a significant increase from past years.

Prevalence by Ethnicity

Research indicates that the prevalence of ED varies by ethnicity, although the reasons for this are not entirely understood and may involve a complex interplay of genetic, environmental, and lifestyle factors.

- Caucasian Men: Studies suggest that Caucasian men have a moderate prevalence rate, ranging from 20-40% depending on age and other risk factors.

- **African American Men:** Some studies indicate a slightly higher prevalence among African American men, although more research is needed to confirm these findings.
- **Asian Men:** Lower prevalence rates have been reported in some Asian populations, but again, more research is needed to provide a comprehensive view.

The Importance of Seeking Medical Advice

In today's age of information, it's easier than ever to search for health-related information online. While the internet is a valuable resource for learning, it should not replace professional medical advice. The importance of seeking medical advice from qualified healthcare providers cannot be overstated. This article aims to explore why consulting a healthcare professional is crucial for accurate diagnosis, effective treatment, and overall well-being.

Why Self-Diagnosis is Risky

The internet is flooded with medical information, and it's tempting to self-diagnose based on symptoms you read about online. However, self-diagnosis can be incredibly risky for several reasons:

1. Inaccurate Information: Not all sources are reliable, and misinformation can lead to incorrect self-diagnosis and inappropriate treatment.
2. Complexity of Medical Conditions: Many symptoms are common to multiple conditions, and only a healthcare provider can accurately diagnose and treat you.
3. Risk of Complications: Without professional guidance, you may overlook serious conditions or complications that require immediate attention.
4. Psychological Stress: Self-diagnosis can also lead to unnecessary stress and anxiety, which can exacerbate symptoms.

The Role of Healthcare Providers

Healthcare providers undergo years of education and training to diagnose and treat medical conditions effectively. They can:

1. Provide Accurate Diagnosis: Through physical examinations, medical history, and diagnostic tests, healthcare providers can offer a more accurate diagnosis than you can achieve on your own.
2. Offer Tailored Treatment: Treatment is often personalized based on your medical history,

current condition, and other factors that only a healthcare provider can evaluate.

3. Monitor Progress: Regular check-ups allow healthcare providers to monitor your condition and adjust treatment as necessary.

4. Provide Emotional Support: Dealing with health issues can be emotionally taxing. Healthcare providers can offer emotional support and guide you through the treatment process.

When to Seek Medical Advice

1. Persistent Symptoms: If you experience symptoms that persist for an extended period, it's crucial to consult a healthcare provider.

2. Severe Symptoms: Any severe symptoms, such as extreme pain, difficulty breathing, or sudden changes in vision or mobility, require immediate medical attention.

3. Chronic Conditions: If you have a chronic condition like diabetes, hypertension, or heart disease, regular medical check-ups are essential for effective management.

4. Preventive Care: Regular screenings and check-ups can help catch potential issues before they become severe problems.

Chapter 1: Understanding Impotence

1.1: What is Impotence?

Impotence, commonly referred to as erectile dysfunction (ED), is a medical condition characterized by the inability to achieve or maintain an erection sufficient for sexual intercourse. While occasional episodes of erectile dysfunction are not uncommon and can be due to various transient factors like stress or fatigue, persistent issues may indicate a more serious underlying condition that requires medical attention.

Types of Impotence

- **Primary Impotence:** This is a rare form where a man has never been able to achieve an erection. It is often due to a congenital or psychological issue.
- **Secondary Impotence:** This is far more common and refers to the condition where a man has had erections before but is currently unable to achieve or maintain them. This can be due to a variety of factors, including psychological issues, medical conditions, or the side effects of medication.

Causes

Impotence can be caused by a variety of factors, which can generally be categorized as follows:

- **Psychological Causes:** Stress, anxiety, depression, and relationship issues can all contribute to impotence. Psychological counseling may be recommended in these cases.
- **Physical Causes:** Conditions like diabetes, hypertension, heart disease, and hormonal imbalances can lead to impotence. Neurological issues and certain surgeries can also cause ED.
- **Lifestyle Factors:** Smoking, excessive alcohol consumption, and drug abuse can contribute to erectile dysfunction. Obesity and a lack of physical exercise are also known risk factors.
- **Medications:** Some medications, including certain antidepressants, antihypertensives, and antihistamines, can cause impotence as a side effect.

Psychological vs. Physical Causes

Erectile dysfunction (ED), or impotence, can be caused by a variety of factors that can generally be categorized into two main types: psychological and physical. Understanding the underlying cause of ED is crucial for effective treatment. Here's a breakdown of psychological vs. physical causes:

Psychological Causes

- *Stress:* Stressful situations can interfere with the body's natural response to sexual stimulation, leading to ED.
- *Anxiety:* Performance anxiety, in particular, can create a cycle of ongoing ED. The more a man experiences ED, the more anxious he may become, which can exacerbate the issue.
- *Depression:* A reduced interest in sexual activity is a common symptom of depression. Some antidepressant medications can also cause ED.
- *Relationship Issues:* Emotional or relational factors can contribute to ED. Lack of emotional intimacy or unresolved conflict can affect sexual function.
- *Psychological Trauma:* Past sexual abuse or other traumatic experiences can also contribute to erectile dysfunction.

Physical Causes

Cardiovascular Disease: Poor heart health can limit blood flow to the penis, making it difficult to achieve an erection.

- *Diabetes:* High levels of blood sugar can damage blood vessels and nerves, including those that stimulate the penis.
- *Hormonal Imbalance:* Low levels of testosterone can affect both libido and the ability to achieve an erection.
- *Neurological Disorders:* Conditions like Parkinson's disease, multiple sclerosis, and stroke can interfere with the nervous system, affecting sexual function.
- *Medications:* Some medications, including certain antihypertensives, antihistamines, and antidepressants, can cause ED as a side effect.
- *Lifestyle Factors:* Smoking, excessive alcohol consumption, and drug abuse can also contribute to ED. Obesity and lack of physical exercise are known risk factors as well.

Diagnosis and Treatment

Diagnosis typically involves a thorough medical history, a physical examination, and sometimes, additional tests like blood tests or imaging studies. Treatment can vary widely depending on the underlying cause and may include:

- **Oral Medications:** Drugs like sildenafil (Viagra), tadalafil (Cialis), and vardenafil (Levitra) are commonly prescribed.
- **Lifestyle Changes:** Diet and exercise can play a significant role in improving erectile function, particularly when the ED is related to cardiovascular health.
- **Psychological Counseling:** If the impotence is due to psychological factors, counseling or sex therapy may be recommended.
- **Other Treatments:** In some cases, vacuum erection devices, intracavernosal injections, or surgical implants may be considered.

It's crucial to consult a healthcare provider for an accurate diagnosis and appropriate treatment plan tailored to your needs.

1.2: Risk Factors

Erectile dysfunction (ED), or impotence, can be influenced by a variety of risk factors that range from lifestyle choices to medical conditions. Understanding these risk factors can help in both prevention and treatment. Here are some of the key risk factors associated with ED:

Age

One of the most significant risk factors for ED is age. While ED can affect men at any age, the likelihood increases significantly with age. For example, the prevalence rises to approximately 40% in men aged 40 and above and can be as high as 60-70% for men over 60.

Medical Conditions

- *Cardiovascular Disease:* Conditions like hypertension and atherosclerosis can impair blood flow, which is essential for an erection.
- *Diabetes:* High blood sugar levels can damage blood vessels and nerves, affecting erectile function.
- *Hormonal Imbalances:* Conditions like hypogonadism can lead to low levels of testosterone, affecting both libido and erectile function.

Lifestyle Factors

- *Smoking:* Tobacco use can restrict blood flow and contribute to atherosclerosis, both of which can lead to ED.
- *Alcohol and Substance Abuse:* Excessive alcohol consumption and substance abuse

can lead to both short-term and long-term ED.

- *Obesity:* Excess weight is associated with conditions like diabetes and cardiovascular disease, which can lead to ED.
- *Lack of Physical Activity:* A sedentary lifestyle can increase the risk of developing conditions that contribute to ED.

Psychological Factors

Stress and Anxiety: These can interfere with the body's natural response to sexual stimulation.

Depression: This can reduce interest in sexual activity, and some antidepressant medications can also cause ED.

Relationship Issues: Emotional or relational factors can contribute to ED. Lack of emotional intimacy or unresolved conflict can affect sexual function.

Medications

Certain medications can have ED as a side effect. These may include:

- Antidepressants: Particularly selective serotonin reuptake inhibitors (SSRIs).

- Antihypertensives: Such as beta-blockers.
- Antihistamines: Some over-the-counter antihistamines can cause temporary ED.

Other Factors

- *Surgery and Medical Treatments:* Procedures affecting the pelvic area or spinal cord can cause ED.
- *Chronic Illness:* Conditions like chronic kidney disease can also contribute to ED.

Understanding these risk factors can help individuals take preventive measures and seek appropriate treatment. If you experience symptoms of ED, it's crucial to consult a healthcare provider for an accurate diagnosis and tailored treatment plan.

1.3: The Psychological Impact

Erectile dysfunction (ED), commonly known as impotence, is often viewed primarily as a physical condition. While the physiological aspects of ED are undoubtedly important, the psychological impact of the condition is frequently overlooked. This essay aims to delve into the emotional and psychological repercussions of ED, exploring how it affects self-esteem, relationships, and mental well-being.

The Stigma Surrounding ED

The societal stigma surrounding erectile dysfunction often exacerbates the psychological toll it takes on individuals. Men may feel emasculated or less "manly" due to their inability to perform sexually, which can lead to feelings of shame or inadequacy. The stigma can also deter men from seeking medical advice, further perpetuating the cycle of anxiety and dysfunction.

Impact on Self-Esteem

One of the most immediate psychological impacts of ED is on a man's self-esteem. The ability to achieve and maintain an erection is often linked, albeit erroneously, to virility and masculinity. When this ability is compromised, it can lead to a damaging self-perception. Men may feel inadequate or less competent, not just in the sexual sphere but in other areas of life as well.

Strain on Relationships

Erectile dysfunction doesn't just affect the individual; it also has a significant impact on romantic relationships. The inability to engage in satisfying sexual activity can create tension between partners. It can lead to a decline in intimacy and may even cause partners to question the stability and future of the relationship. The psychological stress can also extend to the partner, who may feel unattractive or inadequate, wrongly believing themselves to be the cause of the issue.

Mental Health Implications

The psychological impact of ED can extend to broader mental health issues. Chronic stress and anxiety related to sexual performance can lead to conditions like depression. In some cases, the mental health impact can become severe enough to require medication, which can, in turn, exacerbate ED, creating a vicious cycle.

The Importance of Holistic Treatment

Given the profound psychological impact of ED, a holistic approach to treatment is crucial. Alongside medical interventions like medication or surgery, psychological counseling can offer significant benefits. Cognitive-behavioral therapy (CBT) and couples counseling can help address the emotional and relational aspects of ED. Lifestyle changes, such as exercise and stress management techniques, can also help improve both physical and mental well-being.

Chapter 2: Treatment Options
2.1: Lifestyle Changes

In the modern era, the rapid pace of life, technological advancements, and urbanization have drastically altered the way we live. While these changes have brought about numerous conveniences, they have also introduced a myriad of health challenges. From sedentary habits to unhealthy diets, the modern lifestyle has become synonymous with various health risks. However, the solution to many of these problems lies in the very cause: lifestyle changes. This essay delves into the transformative power of lifestyle modifications and their profound impact on holistic well-being.

Lifestyle changes are often recommended as the first line of defense against many health conditions. Whether it's cardiovascular diseases, diabetes, or mental health disorders, a shift in daily habits can significantly alter the course of these conditions. But what does it mean to change one's lifestyle, and why is it so impactful?

Firstly, our daily habits, from what we eat to how often we move, play a pivotal role in determining our overall health. Consuming a diet rich in processed foods, sugars, and unhealthy fats can lead to weight gain, increased cholesterol, and heightened risk of diseases. On the other hand, a balanced diet, replete with whole grains, lean proteins, and plenty of fruits and vegetables, can boost immunity, improve metabolism, and reduce the risk of chronic diseases.

Physical activity is another cornerstone of a healthy lifestyle. In an age where many work hours seated at desks and rely on vehicles for even short distances, physical inactivity has become a silent epidemic. Incorporating regular exercise, be it brisk walking, yoga, or more intensive workouts, can improve cardiovascular health, enhance mood, and increase longevity.

Beyond diet and exercise, lifestyle changes also encompass mental and emotional well-being. Prioritizing mental health, managing stress, and ensuring adequate sleep are all integral to a holistic lifestyle. Practices like meditation, journaling, or even simple breathing exercises can significantly reduce stress, improve focus, and contribute to emotional equilibrium.

However, while the benefits of lifestyle changes are well-documented, implementing them is often challenging. It requires commitment, consistency, and often, a shift in mindset. The modern world is filled with temptations, from fast food to binge-watching TV shows. Overcoming these temptations and making conscious choices every day is the key to successful lifestyle modification.

2.2: Medical Treatments

While lifestyle changes and psychological counseling can be effective in treating some cases, medical treatments are often required for persistent or severe ED. This essay aims to provide a comprehensive guide to the various medical treatments available for erectile dysfunction.

Oral Medications

Oral medications are often the first line of treatment for erectile dysfunction. The most commonly prescribed are phosphodiesterase type 5 (PDE5) inhibitors, which include:

1. Sildenafil (Viagra)
2. Tadalafil (Cialis)
3. Vardenafil (Levitra)

These medications work by enhancing the effects of nitric oxide, a chemical that relaxes muscles in the penis, allowing for increased blood flow during sexual arousal. It's important to note that these medications do not produce an erection without sexual stimulation.

Injections and Suppositories

For men who cannot take oral medications or find them ineffective, alternative treatments like injections and suppositories are available. Alprostadil is a medication that can be injected directly into the penis or inserted as a pellet in the urethra, leading to an erection. While effective, these methods are generally considered less convenient than oral medications.

Vacuum Erection Devices

Vacuum erection devices, also known as penis pumps, are mechanical devices that create a vacuum around the penis, drawing blood into it and causing an erection. A constriction ring is then placed at the base of the penis to maintain the erection. This method is often used when medication is not suitable or effective.

Surgical Options

In severe cases where other treatments have failed, surgical options may be considered. These include:

- Penile Implants: These are devices implanted into the penis, allowing for a controlled erection.
- Vascular Surgery: This is a more complex procedure aimed at improving blood flow to the penis.

It's important to note that surgical options are generally considered a last resort due to the risks and complications involved.

Hormone Therapy

In some cases, erectile dysfunction may be caused by hormonal imbalances. Testosterone replacement therapy can be an effective treatment in these cases. However, it's crucial to undergo thorough medical evaluation to determine whether hormone therapy is appropriate.

2.3: Alternative Therapies

While medical treatments like oral medications and surgical interventions are widely used, some individuals turn to alternative therapies for various reasons, including side effects, contraindications, or personal preference. This essay explores some of the alternative therapies available for treating erectile dysfunction.

Herbal Remedies

Various herbal remedies claim to improve sexual function and have been used for centuries in different cultures. Some of the most commonly cited include:

1. Ginseng: Often referred to as "herbal Viagra," ginseng is believed to improve

erectile function, although scientific evidence is limited.

2. Yohimbe: Derived from the bark of an African tree, yohimbe has been shown to be effective in some studies, but it can have significant side effects, including high blood pressure and anxiety.

3. L-arginine: This amino acid is thought to improve blood flow and has been studied as a potential treatment for ED, often in combination with other substances like pycnogenol.

Acupuncture

Acupuncture involves inserting thin needles into specific points on the body and has been used to treat a variety of conditions, including ED. While some studies suggest that acupuncture can improve erectile function, the evidence is not strong enough to conclusively recommend this as a reliable treatment.

Dietary Changes

While not a standalone treatment for ED, dietary changes can complement other treatments. A diet rich in fruits, vegetables, whole grains, and fish, and with fewer servings of red meat and refined grains, may reduce the risk of ED.

Physical Therapy

Pelvic floor exercises, often referred to as Kegel exercises, can help strengthen the muscles involved in achieving and maintaining an erection. Physical therapy can be an effective treatment for ED, especially when the condition is caused by physical factors like surgery or trauma.

Chapter 3: Introduction to Cialis Tadalafil

3.1: What is Cialis Tadalafil?

Cialis Tadalafil is an oral medication commonly used to treat erectile dysfunction (ED) in men. It belongs to a class of drugs known as phosphodiesterase type 5 (PDE5) inhibitors, which also includes other medications like sildenafil (Viagra) and vardenafil (Levitra). Tadalafil is also approved for the treatment of benign prostatic hyperplasia (BPH), a condition characterized by an enlarged prostate that can cause urinary symptoms.

Mechanism of Action

Cialis Tadalafil works by inhibiting the action of the enzyme phosphodiesterase type 5 (PDE5). This enzyme is responsible for breaking down cyclic guanosine monophosphate (cGMP), a substance that plays a crucial role in achieving and maintaining an erection. By inhibiting PDE5, Tadalafil allows cGMP to remain active for a longer period, thus facilitating an erection in the presence of sexual stimulation.

Side Effects and Precautions

Like all medications, Cialis Tadalafil comes with potential side effects, which may include:

- Headache
- Flushing
- Indigestion
- Back pain
- Muscle aches

More severe but rare side effects include sudden vision loss, hearing loss, and priapism—an erection that lasts more than four hours and requires immediate medical attention.

It's essential to consult a healthcare provider before starting Cialis Tadalafil, especially if you have a history of heart problems, are taking nitrates, or have other medical conditions that may interact with the medication.

3.2: Advantages Over Other Treatments

Cialis Tadalafil offers several advantages over other treatment options for erectile dysfunction (ED), making it a popular choice for many men. Here are some of the key benefits:

Long Duration of Action

One of the most significant advantages of Cialis Tadalafil is its extended duration of action. Unlike other PDE5 inhibitors like sildenafil (Viagra) and vardenafil (Levitra), which generally last for about 4 to 6 hours, a single dose of Cialis can remain effective for up to 36 hours. This long-lasting effect provides a larger window of opportunity for sexual activity, allowing for greater spontaneity and less need for planning. This is particularly beneficial for men who engage in sexual activity more than once within a 36-hour period, as they don't need to take multiple doses.

Flexibility in Dosing

Cialis offers flexibility in dosing that is not commonly found in other ED medications. It can be taken as needed before sexual activity, or at a lower dose on a daily basis for those who are more sexually active. This daily dosing option not only allows for spontaneous sexual activity but also may help improve urinary symptoms in men who have benign prostatic hyperplasia (BPH) in addition to ED.

Lower Side Effect Profile

While all medications come with potential side effects, many users find that Cialis Tadalafil has fewer or more tolerable side effects compared to other ED medications. For example, it is less likely to cause visual disturbances, a side effect sometimes reported with sildenafil. The side effects that do occur, such as headache or muscle aches, are generally mild and may diminish with continued use.

Versatility in Treating Co-Existing Conditions

Cialis Tadalafil is also approved for the treatment of benign prostatic hyperplasia (BPH), a condition that can cause urinary symptoms like difficulty in starting urination or frequent urination. For men who suffer from both ED and BPH, Cialis offers a two-in-one treatment approach, addressing both conditions simultaneously. This can be particularly convenient and cost-effective for patients.

Easier to Integrate into Lifestyle

Because of its long duration of action and flexibility in dosing, many men find it easier to integrate Cialis into their lifestyles compared to other ED treatments. There's less need to time the medication around meals or avoid certain foods, as it is effective regardless of food intake. This makes it a more practical option for many men, especially those with busy or unpredictable schedules.

Chapter 4: How to Use Cialis Tadalafil
4.1: Dosage

One of the key advantages Cialis Tadalafil offers is flexibility in terms of dosing. Understanding the various dosage options and how they should be administered can help ensure the medication's effectiveness while minimizing potential side effects.

Cialis Tadalafil is typically available in tablet form, with dosages ranging from 2.5 mg to 20 mg. The tablets are almond-shaped and come in various sizes and colors, depending on the dosage.

Dosage for Erectile Dysfunction

1. *As-Needed Basis:* For those who plan to engage in sexual activity but not regularly, Cialis can be taken on an as-needed basis. The recommended starting dose is usually 10 mg, taken at least 30 minutes before sexual activity. Depending on the effectiveness and any side effects, the dose can be adjusted up to 20 mg or down to 5 mg.
2. *Daily Use:* For men who engage in sexual activity more than twice a week, Cialis offers a daily dosing option. The recommended starting dose for daily use is 2.5 mg, taken at

approximately the same time every day, without regard to the timing of sexual activity. The dose may be increased to 5 mg based on efficacy and tolerability.

Dosage for Benign Prostatic Hyperplasia (BPH)

For treating BPH symptoms, the recommended dose is 5 mg once a day. This dosage is also effective for men who have both BPH and ED, providing a dual benefit.

Special Populations

1. *Older Adults:* Older men may be more sensitive to the effects of Cialis Tadalafil. Therefore, a lower starting dose may be considered, and adjustments should be made cautiously.
2. *Liver or Kidney Impairment:* For patients with liver or kidney issues, the medication may stay in the system longer, requiring dosage adjustments. It's crucial to consult a healthcare provider for personalized recommendations.
3. *Drug Interactions:* If you are taking medications that interact with Cialis, such as certain antihypertensives or antifungals, your healthcare provider may adjust your Cialis dosage or recommend an alternative treatment.

Precautions

1. *Timing:* While Cialis is known for its long-lasting effects, it's essential to take it at least 30 minutes before sexual activity when used on an as-needed basis.
2. *Food Interactions:* One of the benefits of Cialis is that it can be taken with or without food. However, excessive alcohol consumption should be avoided as it can increase the risk of side effects.
3. *Overdose:* Taking more than the recommended dose can lead to severe side effects or complications. In case of a suspected overdose, seek medical attention immediately.

4.2: Timing

When it comes to medications like Cialis Tadalafil, timing can be a crucial factor in determining the drug's effectiveness. Understanding the optimal timing for taking Cialis can help maximize its benefits while minimizing potential side effects. This article aims to provide an in-depth look at the various timing considerations for Cialis Tadalafil.

Timing for As-Needed Use

For men who use Cialis on an as-needed basis for ED, the timing is particularly important. The medication should be taken at least 30 minutes before planned sexual activity. This allows sufficient time for the drug to be absorbed into the bloodstream and exert its effect. Given that the effects of Cialis can last up to 36 hours, this provides a large window for sexual spontaneity, making it less necessary to time the medication to the exact minute of planned sexual activity.

Timing for Daily Use

For those who opt for the daily dosage option, consistency in timing is key. Taking the medication at the same time each day can help maintain a constant level of the drug in your system, which can be beneficial for both ED and BPH symptoms. Whether you choose to take it in the morning or at night, sticking to a schedule can enhance the medication's effectiveness.

Timing and Food Intake

One of the advantages of Cialis over other ED medications is that it can be taken with or without food. However, it's worth noting that a very fatty meal could slow down the medication's absorption, potentially delaying its effects. While this is generally not a significant concern, for men who are looking for quicker onset of effects, taking the medication on an empty stomach or after a light meal might be preferable.

Timing and Alcohol Consumption

While moderate alcohol consumption is generally considered safe when taking Cialis, excessive alcohol use should be avoided. Alcohol can lower blood pressure, and combining it with Cialis may enhance this effect, potentially leading to dizziness or fainting. If you plan to consume alcohol, it's best to do so in moderation and preferably well before or after taking Cialis.

Timing and Other Medications

If you're taking other medications, especially those that might interact with Cialis, the timing can become more complicated. For example, medications like nitrates, commonly used for chest pain, can interact dangerously with Cialis, leading to a significant drop in blood pressure. Always consult a healthcare provider to ensure that it's safe to take Cialis with any other medications you're using.

Timing and Special Populations

For older adults or those with liver or kidney impairments, the medication may stay in the system longer. This could mean that the timing of the medication needs to be adjusted to prevent potential side effects. Consultation with a healthcare provider is essential for personalized timing recommendations in these cases.

4.3: Contraindications

While it is generally well-tolerated and effective for these conditions, there are certain situations where its use is contraindicated. Understanding these contraindications is crucial for ensuring the safe and effective use of the medication. Here's what you need to know:

Contraindication with Nitrates

One of the most significant contraindications for Cialis is the use of nitrates, which are medications commonly used to treat angina or chest pain. Combining Cialis with nitrates can lead to a dangerous drop in blood pressure, which could result in fainting, stroke, or heart attack.

Contraindication with Certain Blood Pressure Medications

Alpha-blockers, often used to treat high blood pressure or an enlarged prostate, can also interact dangerously with Cialis. This combination can lead to a significant drop in blood pressure, especially when standing up from a sitting or lying position, which could lead to dizziness or fainting.

Severe Liver or Kidney Disease

Patients with severe liver or kidney disease are generally advised not to take Cialis. The medication is metabolized in the liver and excreted through the kidneys, and impaired function of these organs could lead to increased levels of the drug in the bloodstream, heightening the risk of side effects.

Recent Heart Attack or Stroke

If you've had a heart attack or stroke within the last six months, the use of Cialis is generally contraindicated. The medication can put additional strain on the heart, which could be dangerous in these situations.

Hypotension

Cialis is contraindicated for individuals with low blood pressure (hypotension). The medication can further lower blood pressure, which could lead to symptoms like dizziness, fainting, and in severe cases, shock.

Allergic Reactions

If you have had an allergic reaction to Cialis or any of its ingredients in the past, you should avoid the medication. Allergic reactions can range from mild symptoms like itching and rash to more severe symptoms like difficulty breathing or swelling of the face, lips, or tongue.

Other Medications

Certain other medications, such as some antifungals and HIV protease inhibitors, can interact with Cialis, leading to increased levels of the drug in the bloodstream. While not strictly a contraindication, this interaction may require dose adjustments or alternative treatments.

Chapter 5: Side Effects and Complications

5.1: Common Side Effects

While Cialis Tadalafil is generally well-tolerated, like all medications, it comes with a range of potential side effects. Understanding these side effects can help you manage them effectively and know when to seek medical attention. Here are some of the most common side effects associated with Cialis Tadalafil:

Headache

One of the most frequently reported side effects of Cialis is headache. While generally mild, headaches can be bothersome for some users. Over-the-counter pain relievers like acetaminophen or ibuprofen can often alleviate this symptom. Drinking plenty of water may also help.

Indigestion or Heartburn

Some users experience indigestion or heartburn after taking Cialis. Antacids can usually provide quick relief for these symptoms. Eating a smaller meal before taking the medication may also help minimize digestive issues.

Back Pain and Muscle Aches

Cialis can sometimes cause back pain or muscle aches, typically between 12 to 24 hours after taking the medication. These symptoms usually go away within 48 hours. Over-the-counter pain relievers and warm baths may help alleviate these symptoms.

Flushing

Facial flushing or redness is another common side effect. This is usually temporary and tends to diminish on its own. Staying in a cool environment and avoiding alcohol can help manage flushing.

Nasal Congestion

Some users report experiencing nasal congestion when taking Cialis. Over-the-counter decongestants or saline nasal sprays can often provide relief.

Dizziness

While less common, some people may experience dizziness, especially when standing up from a sitting or lying position. If you experience this, it's advisable to sit or lie down until the symptom passes and to rise slowly when standing up.

Vision Changes

Though rare, some users have reported changes in vision, including a bluish tint or difficulty distinguishing between blue and green. If you experience any vision changes, it's crucial to consult a healthcare provider immediately.

5.2: What to Do in Case of Side Effects

Knowing what to do if you experience side effects can help you manage them effectively and ensure your safety. Here's a practical guide on what steps to take.

Mild Side Effects

Headache

- Over-the-counter pain relievers like acetaminophen or ibuprofen can often alleviate headaches.
- Drinking plenty of water may also help.

Indigestion or Heartburn

- Antacids can usually provide quick relief.
- Consider eating a smaller meal before taking the medication to minimize digestive issues.

Back Pain and Muscle Aches

- Over-the-counter pain relievers and warm baths may help alleviate these symptoms.
- If the pain persists for more than 48 hours, consult a healthcare provider.

Flushing

- Staying in a cool environment and avoiding alcohol can help manage flushing.

Nasal Congestion

- Over-the-counter decongestants or saline nasal sprays can often provide relief.

Moderate to Severe Side Effects

Dizziness

- Sit or lie down until the symptom passes.
- Rise slowly when standing up.
- If dizziness persists or worsens, consult a healthcare provider.

Vision Changes

- If you experience any vision changes, such as a bluish tint or difficulty distinguishing between colors, seek medical attention immediately.

Hearing Loss

- Sudden hearing loss is a rare but serious side effect. If this occurs, stop taking Cialis and seek emergency medical care.

Emergency Situations

Priapism

- An erection lasting more than four hours is a medical emergency and requires immediate attention to prevent long-term damage.

Severe Hypotension

- A significant drop in blood pressure can be life-threatening. If you experience symptoms like extreme dizziness, fainting, or chest pain, seek emergency medical care.

General Guidelines

1. Consult a Healthcare Provider: If you experience any side effects, it's always a good idea to consult a healthcare provider for personalized advice.
2. Discontinue Use: For severe or alarming side effects, stop taking the medication and seek medical attention immediately.
3. Review Other Medications: Make sure to inform your healthcare provider about any other medications you're taking, as the side effects could be due to drug interactions.
4. Follow Prescribed Guidelines: Always take the medication as prescribed, and do not exceed the recommended dosage without consulting a healthcare provider.

Chapter 6: Frequently Asked Questions

Can women take Cialis Tadalafil?

Cialis Tadalafil is not approved for use in women and should not be used for treating sexual dysfunction in women. The medication is specifically formulated to treat erectile dysfunction and benign prostatic hyperplasia in men.

Can I take Cialis Tadalafil if I don't have ED or BPH?

Cialis Tadalafil should only be taken for medical conditions for which it is prescribed. Using it recreationally or without a healthcare provider's guidance can lead to adverse effects and make it difficult to diagnose any underlying conditions that may require treatment.

Is it safe to take Cialis Tadalafil with herbal supplements for ED?

The safety of taking Cialis Tadalafil with herbal supplements for ED has not been well-studied. Some herbal supplements can interact with prescription medications and may increase the risk of side effects. Always consult a healthcare provider before combining Cialis with any other medications or supplements.

Can I split Cialis Tadalafil tablets to lower the dose?

Cialis tablets are not scored, meaning they are not designed to be split. Splitting the tablets can result in uneven doses, which may reduce effectiveness or increase the risk of side effects. If you require a lower dose, consult your healthcare provider for an appropriate prescription.

How long does it take for Cialis Tadalafil to start working?

Cialis Tadalafil generally starts working within 30 to 60 minutes when taken on an as-needed basis. However, the time can vary depending on individual factors like metabolism, age, and whether you've eaten a large meal.

Can I take Cialis Tadalafil if I'm also taking anticoagulants?

Cialis Tadalafil does not have a direct interaction with anticoagulants like warfarin. However, if you're taking anticoagulants, it's crucial to consult a healthcare provider before starting Cialis, as other medical conditions or medications you're taking may pose risks.

Does Cialis Tadalafil affect fertility?

There is no evidence to suggest that Cialis Tadalafil affects fertility in men. The medication is designed to treat erectile dysfunction and benign prostatic hyperplasia and has not been shown to impact sperm quality or fertility.

Can I take Cialis Tadalafil more than once a day?

For most patients, the recommended starting dose of Cialis for as-needed use is 10 mg per day, and for daily use, it's 2.5 mg. Taking more than the recommended dose without a healthcare provider's guidance can increase the risk of side effects and is generally not advised.

Is it safe to buy Cialis Tadalafil online?

While it may be convenient to buy Cialis online, it's crucial to ensure that you're purchasing from a reputable source. Counterfeit medications can be ineffective or even harmful. Always look for online pharmacies that require a prescription and are accredited by relevant authorities.

Printed in Great Britain
by Amazon

40965200R00026